The
Whole Body
Breathing

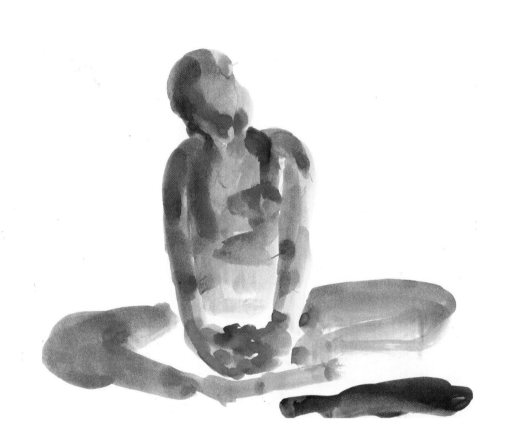

The Whole Body Breathing

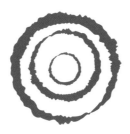

Discovering the subtle
rhythms of yoga

Sandra Sabatini & Michal Havkin

Watercolours by Orly Maiberg

YOGAWORDS

First published in 2018 by YogaWords, an imprint of Pinter and Martin Ltd

Text copyright © Sandra Sabatini and Michal Havkin 2018
Watercolours copyright © Orly Maiberg

ISBN 978-1-906756-55-0

Managing Editor: Zoë Blanc
Editor: Jan Heron
Design: Blok Graphic, London

A catalogue record for this book is available from the British library.

Printed in the EU by Hussar

Pinter and Martin Ltd
6 Effra Parade
London SW2 1PS

pinterandmartin.com/yogawords

YOGAWORDS

To Vanda who encouraged us to
search with curiosity and playfulness

Acknowledgements

Our deepest gratitude goes to our teachers for having inspired us and shown us the way as well as to our students for welcoming our attempts to transform experiences into clear words. To our children, grandchildren, family and friends. Without your love and constant support we wouldn't keep finding our way back onto our yoga mats. Thank you.

To Martin, Maria, Zoë Blanc and Zoë Hutton for their professional support and care in creating this book. To Jan Heron for turning the first draft into a more clear and approachable text. To Orly for generously allowing us to use drawings from her collection, and for having been artistically at our sides all along. To Aviva, Bo and Carolin for providing us the best of places to practise, sit and write quietly.

Contents

Foreword

This book provides a reminder of a pattern of daily practice. The practice helps remind the body of its capacity to adapt and receive breath and sense gravity. This small book provides guiding questions to encourage us to begin to experience for ourselves how our body can breathe and accept the force of gravity and deploy imagination and intuition.

When we slip out of the onward flow of our lives for a period of the day for practice to sense the ground, and let the breath mingle with the surrounding space, then our bodies become more porous and can cleanse the fixity of the past. These proposals allow us to avoid the unwitting dragging of the past along which burdens us. We let go of the past through our focus on the forces of the breath and gravity on the body in the present.

We may feel refreshed as if by a holiday and able to heed the subtle messages from the body.

The writers have been able to capture the practice of the breath and gravity in the way the Egyptians captured birds alive with nets, not harming them at all. The writers do not preach at us, but let us in on the secrets they have discovered through their learning and practice, and their capacity to listen.

Ann Colcord

Introduction

Preparing each and every workshop is for both of us a laboratory: studying, searching and tuning in to the theme. Teaching becomes a full-size experiment with everyone taking part.

Practising awareness through the various parts of the body is a full body experience: being in total connection with the earth below and the space above.

It becomes real. The spine, from the lowest part to the top is alive and connected. It awakens the whole body to a different placement and alignment. The result is a new body, lighter and taller.

Looking at the students, we can clearly see the vivid change they have been through. Teaching has the same effect on us as teachers.

Following in the footsteps of Vanda Scaravelli's teaching where awareness, breath and freedom are the essential elements, our guidance becomes an everlasting experiment full of joy, insights and love.

Sandra Sabatini & Michal Havkin

A travelling companion

Looking for the place where mind and body meet requires inner spaciousness and infinite time. Every day immerse yourself in the playfulness and fun of the research, not expecting anything. Often what floats up is only a longer breath or the uncovering of a microscopic dormant spot.

So this book is a travelling companion, to take along with you and keep at your side if you feel that at any time the inventiveness is withering away.

Use it in small bites that you can savour and chew until the nourishing parts are fully absorbed.

No need to rush to the following page … wait and repeat the sequence until the whole being digests it.

You are not alone.

Feel that you are supported and guided by wonderful and everlasting friends: your breath, the very earth and the space around you.

Be in touch with the breath, its path and its rhythm, learn to listen to it.

Be in touch with the earth, its offers and demands, learn to listen to it.

Be in touch with the space around and above you, its suggestions and lightness, learn to listen to it.

You are never alone while standing and walking step by step on this ancient road.

At the beginning

At the beginning of our yoga exploration, we may be overburdened with all the impositions connected to the basic postures: sitting, walking and standing.

We have been moulded into a vertical stiffness where we are only capable of holding ourselves upright. In this condition we are constantly struggling against gravity with a false aim of reaching upwards.

It takes a long journey of unwinding to go back to the very primal confidence we had as children when we trusted gravity. Only by sinking back to this natural state will we be able to experience movements which are round and circular.

Like everything else in nature, our bodies move more efficiently and elegantly in curves. We are built in such a way that moving along circular lines brings a deep sense of wellbeing.

The discovery of this gift, given to us by nature, comes when we give ourselves permission to play, explore and drop rigidity. The path of unwinding ahead of us is paved with months and years of meticulous letting go.

And we will soon discover that the most powerful tool given to us is the breath: the exhalation with its cleansing properties and the inhalation with its enriching elements.

Awareness of the natural unfolding movement of the exhalation is the best key to this discovery. Inner spaces will be encouraged to release. Inner organs will soften and the breath itself will be longer and free.

Once we trust our natural breath, the existence of different movements inside and outside the body – movements which are round and spiralling – will dawn on us.

There is a great beauty in contacting these movements, a big surprise in meeting them.

These discoveries are followed by infinite joy and wellbeing. The opportunity for transformation is there.

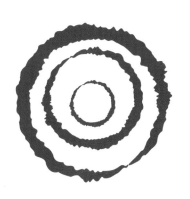

chapter one

The whole body breathing

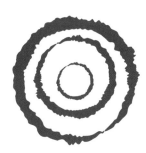

"Like a hollow bamboo
rest at ease in your body"

Yoga of The Mahamudra

The whole body breathing

Our first and most loyal teacher is the earth.

Through touching the earth and being touched by it, we regain the physical sensation of our back, our front and our two sides.

By giving the weight of the body to the earth, we learn to surrender to the external force of gravity. The response from the ground widens and makes more precise our physical sense of the body.

This dialogue with the earth is the source of all our discoveries.

In our daily lives, we keep losing this contact, this link with the earth and it becomes a continual practice to find it again.

Our vision of our bodies is usually very fragmented. This whole practice is about reassembling the scattered pieces into one, wholesome unity. It will take us, step by step, to a fuller and clearer picture of the body.

When we develop this sense of the whole body, there is freedom.

Initial suggestions:
How to convey a sense of the whole body

Step 1

Experience the four sides of the body while contacting the earth.

On your back:
Be aware of all the meeting points between your back and the ground and how the ground moves towards your back, wishing to meet it.

Spend a few minutes deepening this dialogue between your back and the ground.

On your front:
Be aware of all the meeting points between your front and the ground and how the ground moves towards your front, wishing to meet it.

Spend a few minutes deepening this dialogue between your front and the ground.

On each side:
Be aware of all the meeting points between your side and the ground and how the ground moves towards your side, wishing to meet it.

Spend a few minutes deepening this dialogue between your side and the ground.

Step 2

Lying on your back with your arms comfortably away from your body, and your legs wide apart.

Be like a star fish, widely spread at the bottom of the sea.

Exhale down through the palms of your hands and the soles of your feet for a few rounds of breath.

Stay with the breath sliding out through the whole of your body and the in-breath moving in through the whole of your body.

After a few rounds of breath, play with extending your wrists and hands at the end of the exhalation.

Exhale all the way down to your feet, extending both your ankles and heels.

Repeat the same sequence while lying on your front.

Step 3

Lying on your back with your legs extended, bring both your hands to your upper chest and gently add more weight to your hands as you exhale and release gently to welcome in the inhalation.

Repeat this with the hands on your chest a few times.

Move your hands to the floating ribs and again add more weight to your hands accompanying the releasing of air out and soften them to welcome the air in.

Repeat this a few times.

Move your hands to the navel area and increase the weight of your hands as you exhale, and release to receive the new air.

Repeat for a few rounds of breath.

Step 4

Lying on your right side with the knees bent, support your head and place your left hand on your left thigh.

Gently squeeze the air out with your hand as you exhale and gently release your hand to inhale.
Repeat this a few times.

Gradually move your hand to your left hip, the left side of your waistline, the left side of your lower ribs, upper ribs and inside of the armpits.

In each place squeeze as you exhale and release as you receive the new air, softly and gently.

Turn around to lie on your left side and starting from the right thigh, touch and release this side of your body with your right hand in the same places.

Step 5

Lying on your back, breathe through the inner spaces of the whole body.

Exhale and travel through the inner space of your skull,
the inner space of your throat,
the inner space of your right arm and hand,
the inner space of your left arm and hand,
the inner space of your ribcage,
the inner space of your waistline,
the inner space of your pelvis.

Travel through the inner space of your right leg and foot and the inner space of your left leg and foot.

Repeat this journey of accompanying your breath through your inner space a few times.

Imagine the whole body empty and hollow.

As you accompany your breath through the empty body, visualise the spaciousness within.

Step 6

Standing with feet parallel, spread your toes, rock forwards and back, inviting your feet to a more widely spread contact with the ground below.

Play with shifting the weight from one foot to the other, gently finding the centre between the two.

Let your arms move gradually away from the body without introducing strain or struggle.

Drop them and repeat until there is softness and elegance. With arms slightly away and feet widely spread, experiment with this new stance and let the exhalation roll to both hands and down to both feet.

Rest as the breath reaches the ground and expose yourself to the incoming breath.

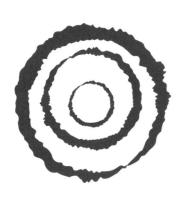

chapter two

Spirals around the spine

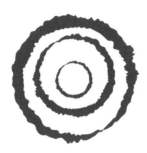

Find your way to the pose by circling
in small, light curves as flies and bees
do when aiming for a definite spot ...

Round movements of spiral gestures
penetrate in depth and can bring
about unexpected results ...

Vanda Scaravelli in *Awakening the Spine*

Spirals around the spine

Allowing the body to move in spirals brings new vitality to the spine, opening and releasing stiff joints and ligaments.

It adds another depth and dimension to our exploration of physicality and awareness.

Inner spaces will be encouraged to widen. Inner organs will soften.

The breath, moving in spirals according to its own nature, will help the whole being towards quietness and receptivity.

A softer and longer breath cycle will follow.

We can induce this natural longing of the body by introducing round movements and subtle curves into our daily practice.

By connecting over and over again the birth of each movement to the spine, there will be less effort and therefore less fatigue. The body's constant wish for suppleness will be granted and integrity will be restored.

Initial suggestions:

Step 1

Standing with feet parallel.

Exhale through both nostrils, following the exhalation towards the horizon.

Inhale, following the inhalation in from the horizon towards you.

Step 2

Standing with feet parallel.

Left arm and hand go to the right shoulder, right arm and hand towards the left hip.

Inhale and exhale in the same way as before, following the path of the breath to and from the horizon.

Swap the position of the hands and repeat.

Step 3

Standing with one foot forward, the body weight evenly divided between the feet.

Left arm and hand go to the right shoulder, right arm and hand towards the left hip.

Inhale and exhale as before, following the breath to and from the horizon.

Swap the position of the hands and repeat.

Step 4

Sitting on the heels.

Hug your body with the arms and hands as you did while standing.

Inhale and exhale following the breath to and from the horizon.

Swap the position of the hands and repeat.

Step 5

Lying on your back.

With the right leg straight, the left knee and thigh move across the right leg in a twist.

Inhale and exhale following the breath towards space and back.

Then change sides.

Step 6

Lying on your back.

With both knees bent, bring your knees and thighs to your chest with an exhalation, and take them to the right side as far as they go without any effort. Let your head roll to the left.

Inhale and exhale following the breath towards space and back.

Then change sides.

Step 7

Sitting and breathing practice. Sit in a comfortable position where you can stay for a few minutes.

Let your hands rest on your knees.

Allow yourself to develop a full inner picture of all sides of the whole spine from the bottom end to the top of it.

Use the exhalation to create space around your spine as if it was being pulled and held by gravity below and the space above.

After a few rounds of breath, allow the exhalation to move in spirals around your spine, repeatedly.

Stay awake and alert for the whole journey of the exhalation from the top of the head to the end of the spine.

Release the hips to gravity and open to receive the inhalation moving in spirals upwards from the earth.

Step 8

Lying on your back with your legs extended.

Surrender to the pull of gravity, let your back widen and listen to your breath for a few minutes.

Roll your head towards the right shoulder and close your right nostril with the index finger of the right hand.

Bend your right knee and place your right foot on the ground. Breathe out and in through the open left nostril, very slowly.

Visualise the exhalation travelling smoothly and gently all the way down your left side in a spiral as far as the foot.

Cleaning, dusting, polishing, rest and be open to receive the inhalation penetrating into the left side of the body.

Keep the right nostril closed all along.

After a few rounds of breath, release the right hand and the right leg. Roll the head to the left and do the same on the other side.

After a few rounds of breath on the left, release the left hand and the left leg. Roll the head back to the centre and breathe from both nostrils for a few rounds.

Play with unfolding the spirals while exhaling through both nostrils.

Realising and lengthening the spirals will come naturally if you give it time.

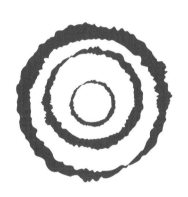

chapter three

Whirlpools along the spine

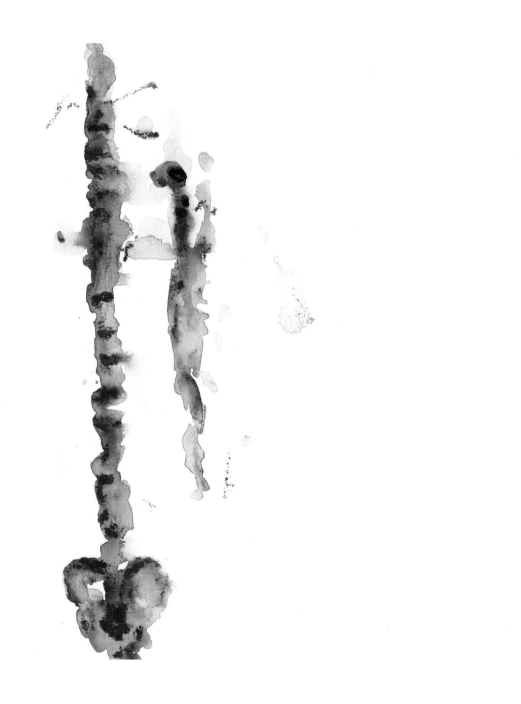

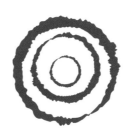

... that state of vulnerability, innocence
and abandon in which, like children,
we are taken by the hand to discover
the kingdom of wonders and marvels,
putting us in touch with nature
where the miracle of existence
is renewed each day.

Vanda Scaravelli in *Awakening the Spine*

Whirlpools along the spine

In this state of intimacy with your breath, its path and discoveries, you are bound to enter and meet powerful places while practising.

Many yoga practitioners have located and explored these special places and named them differently, including chakra, vortex, whirlpool, etc.

We have chosen to protect your own discoveries and carefully avoided labelling these special places you might come across along your spine, as we feel that their coming to life should happen while practising.

At the beginning they are heavily covered with dust and therefore inaccessible.

The state of innocence and stupor are the most likely travelling companions that will lead you by the hand to meet them, one day, unexpectedly.

The proposals you will find in the following pages are assembled to provide you with a completely satisfactory exploration of the special place you are dwelling in.

Enjoy them as a wonderful morning starting place or an evening resting spot.

Through constant daily dusting they start awakening, and the whirlpool in each and every one of them is unfolded and activated.

Stay playful.

Creative.

Open to unexpected sensations and insights.

This is the practice.

The root of being
step by step by step

The tail
folding and unfolding

The navel
home, a dwelling place

The heart
pulsing, pulsing, pulsing

The throat
by the seashore

The eyebrow centre
as captivating as a smile

The crown of the head
breath after breath after breath

The root of being | step by step by step

It is only by exposing the full length of your body to the external pull of gravity below and space above that you can truly experience yourself as a human being.

This simple trusting exposure of the soles of your feet to the earth gives you a sense of belonging that banishes apprehension and secures your place in space on this earth.

Your feet transmit this sense of reliability to the lower part of your legs.

Your knees are asked to soften, introducing a subtle alignment to the opening below.

Your thighs are pulled into this newly awakened sensation of being rebuilt from the earth upwards.

As this physical ripple is allowed to travel upwards, it filters into the pelvis, transmitting microscopic encouragements towards a fully spread-out awareness of the feet, lower legs, knees, upper legs and pelvis.

Your body might give a signal of a new kind of stability, just born.

The first vortex, in the centre of the pelvic floor, is awakening.

Root proposals

A1 | Standing with feet wide apart and parallel.

Spread the soles of your feet from the centre, while exhaling.

Let your body oscillate backwards and forwards.

Exhale as you roll back onto your heels and inhale as you rock forward onto your toes.

Visualise a pendulum, hanging from the base of the spine strengthening your connection to the earth.

A2 | Sitting with legs wide apart.

Shift the weight from one sitting bone to the other and become connected to the vortex in between the two.

Exhale into the space between your two sitting bones and visualise a pendulum spinning into the earth.

Rest and let your breath come from the earth.

A3 | Lying on your back.

Bend your knees up, keeping your feet parallel.

Spread your feet well into the ground.

Send an exhalation down your spine, releasing it between your feet and away from your body.

Let go of your feet and pelvis, and welcome the inhalation.

B1 | Standing with feet parallel.

Place your left foot forward.

Place your arms behind your back and hold the left wrist with your right hand.

Exhale and shift your weight to the back heel and foot, giving space to a whirlpool that moves from the pelvic floor towards the earth.

Inhale and shift your weight to the front foot and toes.

After a few rounds of attentive breath, change the order of the feet and hands.

B2 | Walking slowly, step by step.

Feel the soles of your feet in contact with the ground.

Start walking slowly.

Exhale, spreading the sole of the front foot and its toes, shifting your weight onto it.

Inhale as you slowly peel the back heel off the ground.

B3 | Sitting with the soles of the feet together.

Exhale into the space between your two sitting bones, giving space to a whirlpool, which gathers strength as it gets closer to the earth below.

Your feet receive the very end of the exhalation.

The soles of your feet open, your knees and sitting bones drop.

Rest and receive the in-breath.

B4 | Lying on your back.

Rest your spine with your knees bent and feet parallel to each other on the ground.

After a few rounds of easy natural breath, exhale down one leg and exhale down the other.

As the exhalation unfolds, follow its journey beyond the pelvic floor and away from you.

Rest your feet, legs and pelvis and receive the inhalation.

Root proposals in daily life

While standing:
Visualise your roots crawling into the earth, down through both feet.

While walking:
Feel the difficulties in uprooting the roots underneath your back heel with each and every step.

When sitting:
On a chair, at home, in the office, on the bus, feel fully aware of your sitting bones and the conversation between them and the surface you are sitting on.

Try to sense whether your body weight is equally divided between the two.

Are they both touching the surface they are sitting on in the same way?

At any time of day:
Whenever you can, massage your feet. Open the soles of each foot and extend and elongate each and every toe.

The tail | folding and unfolding

As the effective grip that comes from the earth is allowed to take hold of your feet, legs and hips, the activation of the root of being is naturally followed by the awakening of the tail.

The organic adjustments that come along with this grip induce the pelvis to sway, exposing the tail to microscopic movements.

This constant and clever dialogue with the earth – letting go into it and receiving pulses to grow away from it – adds a sense of inner spaciousness to the pelvis.

The perception of the pelvis changes as confidence in the pull of gravity increases.

Constant and clear attentiveness to the tail will shift the stagnant matter around it, bringing back its original freedom.

In this new-found liveliness, the tail will respond freely to the minute stimulations which crawl from the feet up into the legs and pelvis, into an organism open to listening and receiving them.

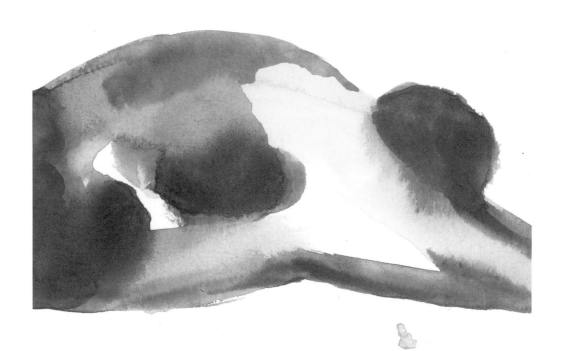

Tail proposals

A1 | Standing with feet parallel.

Place your hands on your hips to help centre the pelvis.

Feel the connection to the ground through your feet and the centre of the pelvic floor.

As you exhale, feel the centre of your pelvic floor get hooked to the ground and your tail widening and elongating.

Rest and wait for the inhalation to come in.

Tail proposals

A2 | Sitting with legs extended and wide apart.

Exhale and release the sitting bones down to the floor.

Let the tail be free to move in between the two sitting bones while keeping your back long and extended.

Exhale and let your back extend forward gradually. Inhale and stay forward and extended.

Exhale again and let your back extend further forward.

Inhale and stay extended forward as you are.

Let the tail be free to sway and swing all along.

Stay forward and extended for a few rounds of breath, giving lots of space and freedom to the tail.

A3 | Lying on your back.

Bend your knees up, keeping your feet parallel on the ground.

Breathe down the spine towards the tail for a few rounds of breath.

Hug your knees gently and let them soften towards your chest.

As you exhale, release and elongate the tail away from you.

Rest and welcome the inhalation.

A4 | Sitting cross-legged.

With your hands, encourage your legs and knees to lengthen towards the ground.

Let your back lean forward.

With each exhalation, lengthen your tail towards the ground and towards the root of being.

Rest and inhale.

With several rounds of breath, gradually come back to sitting upright.

B1 Standing with feet parallel, toes extended.

Place one hand on the pubic bone at the front and the other hand on the tail at the back.

Exhale and gently push yourself backwards towards your heels and release the tail downwards.

Let go and rest.

Now inhale and move gently forward towards your toes.

Play with losing and regaining your balance without falling.

B2 | On all fours.

Slowly fold and unfold the spine.

Move each and every vertebra from the tail to the skull, and vice versa.

Exhale, folding the spine very gently, inwardly.

Rest and inhale, unfolding the spine from the tail up.

B3 | Lying on your back.

Bend your knees up, keeping your feet parallel.

Exhale and watch the exhalation sliding down your spine.

Your feet drop and the tail is lifted slightly off the floor.

Rest with your tail off the ground and watch the breath coming in.

Stay there for a few rounds of breath.

Exhale your back down to the ground and rest.

B4 | Sitting cross-legged.

Slowly exhale and inhale for a few rounds of breath, cleaning the path.

Visualise a golden drop moving down your spine towards your tail, touching each and every vertebra on its way.

Rest and let the in-breath fill up your whole body.

Tail proposals in daily life

While standing or walking:
Place your hands on the region of the tail and rub this area
clockwise and anti-clockwise.

When sitting:
Evenly distribute the weight of your body between the two
sitting bones and reconnect to the space around and below
the tail.

Lying on the ground:
Whenever you can, with the knees bent, place the palm of your
hand under your tail. Stay there for a few rounds of breath,
releasing, widening and resting your tail into your hands.

The navel | home, a dwelling place

When your feet are captured by the magnetism of the earth, the root of being is stimulated to play with this new contact. Your tail enjoys some freshly-discovered freedom and the whole pelvis is searching for a more comfortable place in which to be.

The adjustment to the earth of the pelvis, this voluminous recipient, is accomplished through thousands and thousands of tiny shifts.

It is easily lost, and equally easily regained. Every single event, whether internal or external, is registered by the navel area as major. Absorbing and processing, it is an everlasting task that requires constant attentiveness and acceptance.

The earth below is asking for more stability which will create more lightness above.

Often the lower part of your body lacks weight and consistency, while the upper part is filled with excessive noise. The navel, being the junction between these two worlds, is often overloaded with conflicting stimuli.

The gentle undulation that comes while searching for effortless alignments is a valid tool in activating the navel, which can now clear the excessive noise gathered within it. When time and attentiveness and touch are given to this area, quietness enters and clarity naturally follows. You are home in the dwelling place.

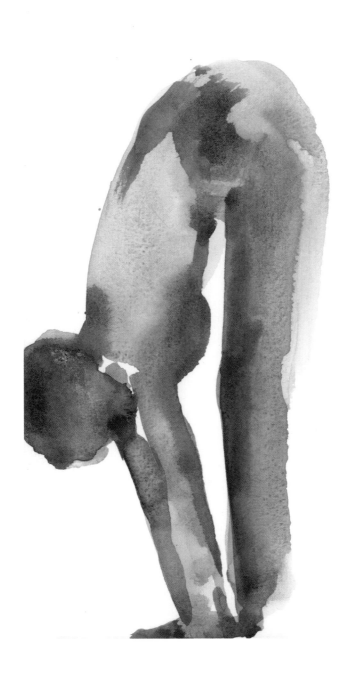

Navel proposals

A1 | Standing with feet parallel.

Place one hand on the navel area and the other on the middle of your waistline at the back.

While exhaling, expose your body to a wave-like movement, which invites the back of your waist to move towards the hand on your back.

Drop the heels, rest and receive the in-breath.

A2 | Lying on your back.

Bend your knees up, keeping your feet parallel.

Bring your hands to your navel and closely follow the journey of your exhalation.

As the breath reaches the navel area, drop the back of your waist to the ground, so that the breath can travel down into your thighs, knees, calves, ankles and feet.

Rest and let the inhalation move in freely.

A3 | Lying on your back.

Position the soles of your feet together and the thighs and knees open.

Open your arms and hands to the sides, at shoulder level, with the palms of the hands facing up.

Exhale, and gradually close one knee above the other.

Allow the exhalation to move from your navel to your tail and the soles of your feet.

Rest there and let the in-breath move in.

Play with turning your head towards your knees and away from them.

Stay there for a few rounds of breath, open the knees again and repeat on the other side.

A4 | Sitting in half lotus.

With one hand on the middle of your back, extend the spine between the earth and space.

As you exhale, visualise a spiral unfolding around your spine.

The whole lower part of your body is pulled down toward the earth.

Your spine lengthens and your navel softens backwards as you gradually turn to one side.

After a few rounds of breath, swap the position of the legs and arm and practise on the other side.

B1 | Standing with feet parallel.

Place one foot forward, with the body weight evenly divided between the two feet.

Invite an oscillation that sets your body free from unnecessary heaviness and stiffness.

Exhale and let your navel be sucked back towards the spine so that your breath will flow unimpeded to your feet and the ground below.

Swap the position of the feet and repeat.

B2 | Lying on your back.

Bend your knees up, keeping your feet parallel.

Exhale, pressing the navel area down and lifting your tail up, ever so slightly.

Inhale and lift the navel off the ground while pressing your tail down to the ground.

Play with these movements, back and forth, for a few rounds of breath.

B3 | Lying on your back.

Hug your knees.

Exhale and listen to the exhalation softening the navel area.

Allow your knees to get a little closer to your chest.

Rest and listen to the inhalation, allowing your knees to move slightly away from you.

Play with these movements for a few rounds of breath.

B4 | Sitting with legs wide apart.

Place your hands at the back of your waist, on the spine.

Let your hands move from the spine at the back to the navel area at the front a few times, back and forth.

Feel your pelvis being drawn down by the earth.

Rest your hands on your knees.

Visualise the exhalation travelling through your inner space in spiralling movements.

Observe it as it gathers strength inside the pelvis.

Let go of the out-breath and the sitting bones.

Rest and welcome the in-breath.

Navel proposals in daily life

When walking:
Slow down your pace and place both hands on the navel area.

When tired:
Lie on your back with your knees bent. Place your hands on the navel area.

Let your hands rise and fall as the breath comes in and goes out.

While standing:
Transform your whole body into a hollow bamboo cane – still green and without knots.

Let your exhalation flow down, and feel your navel moving backwards to allow the breath to reach your feet.

The heart | pulsing, pulsing, pulsing

Continuous alignment transforms your whole being into a receptive organism.

The standing position becomes a versatile instrument for discovery. The softening of the heart is related to the stability of the lower part of your body.

If wobbling, unstable and uncertain of the earth beneath, the heart will shrink in fear and apprehension, losing its natural cheerfulness.

From your feet, which are stabilised by the pull of gravity, the tail learns to wave, amplifying the subtle movements. The navel centre is pulled back into its natural nest, releasing the upper part of your body into freedom.

The relief that follows is immense. And from now on, weight is dropped and accumulated in the lower part of your body while lightness is restored from the waist up.

The journey from the feet up has brought in another powerful element: space.

Travelling through the root, touching the tail, inviting a softness in the navel, space allures with its offers to blend into your whole body.

A physical widening of the heart area will bring a smile around the breastbone.

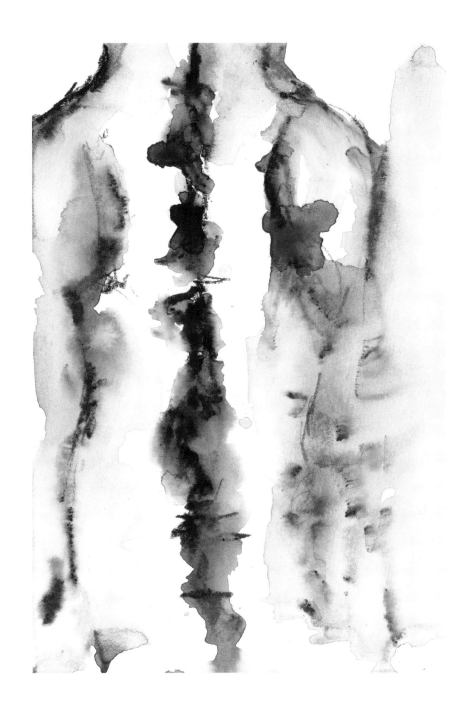

Heart proposals

A1 | Standing with feet parallel.

Place your hands on the sternum and heart area.

Explore the area – the length of it and the shape of the ribs as they move away from it.

Then shift your attention to the right side.

Activate the right foot and extend the right arm above your head.

Investigate the full length of the right side from the heel to the tips of your fingers.

Slowly peel off the other foot from the ground.

Exhale towards your standing heel, rest and inhale all the way up to the tips of your fingers.

After a few rounds of breath, return to the parallel position and move your attention to the left side.

A2 | Standing with feet parallel.

Gently lift one foot off the ground, actively inhaling towards the standing heel, and place it in the opposite inner thigh.

Place your hands next to your heart.

Be willing to adjust to the pull of gravity that comes from the ground, feeling the tiny oscillations.

Consolidate your posture with an exhalation that travels deep into your roots.

As you inhale, your heart brightens up.

After a few rounds of breath, return your foot to the ground and move your attention to the other side.

A3 | Lying on your back.

Bend your knees up, keeping your feet parallel on the ground.

Invite the opening of the heart region with a soft touch of your hands along the sternum ribs.

Listen to the rising and falling of this area as you breathe, encouraging the in-breath to penetrate all hidden corners.

A4 | Sitting in a comfortable position.

Bring the five fingers of your right hand to meet the five fingers of the left. Fingertips simply touch.

Softly place your hands in front of your body at the heart level.

Exhale from an open heart to a soft navel, a long tail down to the root of your being and two sitting bones.

Allow this descending path to gain clarity and vividness.

Allow your pelvis and knees to become heavier into the ground below.

With a more solid connection, now the in-breath will spread more freely and widen your heart.

Enjoy a few minutes of natural deep breathing.

B1 | Standing with feet parallel.

Place one foot forward, with the body weight evenly divided between the two feet.

Place your hands on your breastbone.

After a few breaths, invite your two arms and hands to meet on your back, behind your heart, palms of the hands together.

While exhaling, shift your weight to the back heel.

Let it drop and roll into the ground.

While inhaling, shift your weight forward towards your toes.

Gradually reduce the oscillation and stay in between your two legs and feet, expanding your heart.

B2

Lying on your back.

Bend your knees, keeping your feet parallel.

Invite your hands to the upper part of your chest.

Watch the inhalation as it lifts your collarbones.

They glide upwards and back, bringing a new spaciousness to the heart.

B3

Lying on your back.

Bend your knees, keeping your feet parallel.

As you exhale, invite your feet to open and tail to extend, lifting slightly off the ground.

Soften the navel and let your heart open.

Gradually let this position unfold further, so that your whole back will be slowly lifted off the ground.

Then you can invite your hands to meet behind your back, interlacing all your fingers.

Stay there for a few rounds of breath.

While exhaling, release your hands and arms to the side of your body and bring your back down, one vertebra at a time.

B4 | Sitting with the soles of your feet together.

Allow the knees to open.

Place your two hands on your two feet and exhale with an aum sound, squeezing the feet gently.

Release your feet slightly as you welcome the in-breath.

Repeat this a few times.

Then move your hands to your ankles, your calves, your knees, your thighs, hips, lumbar region and heart.

With each part you touch, stay for a few rounds of breath, squeezing as you exhale and releasing as you inhale.

Heart proposals in daily life

When walking:
Extend your arms and hands to your sides, as if they were as light as wings.

Rotate them inward and outward a few times, inviting the rotation to create an opening in your upper chest and heart.

When sitting:
Bring one hand to your heart area and softly and gently circle the hand around the heart.

When you find yourself sad or heavy:
Bring your hand to your sternum and let your fingers explore the breastbone.

Look for a sagging point along the breastbone and lift it with your fingers, cheering it up.

The throat | by the seashore

Standing becomes an exposure to earth and space that brings various gifts.

The practice of inner alignment is soothing and peace-creating, as it is a well laid-out natural path.

A deep sense of participation unfolds in the whole being; a desire to blend and receive the qualities of the earth and space.

From the waist down, gravity is actively pulling and supporting. From the waist up, space offers all its virtues.

This organic amalgam enhances the awakening of subtle places otherwise dormant.

While the root is asking to be connected to the earth, the tail enjoys its new mobility, the navel touched by awareness rejoices and the heart smiles with levity. And then this cheerfulness around the heart penetrates to the throat.

Space filters into an area often tight and rigid. The delicate and sensitive throat is constantly exposed to inner and outer noise.

Bringing attention to the throat uncovers a need that has been postponed for far too long.

This touch of awareness is a reminder of the importance of silence in our practice and our daily life.

This touch will open a dialogue with the inner voice that can only take place when there is quietness inside.

Space, when gently wrapped around the throat, protects the rhythmical pulsation of the outgoing and incoming breaths. You are reminded of the soothing sound of waves as they reach the shore and retrace back into the vast ocean.

The throat is a gateway of infinite sensitivity – a filter between the head and the heart.

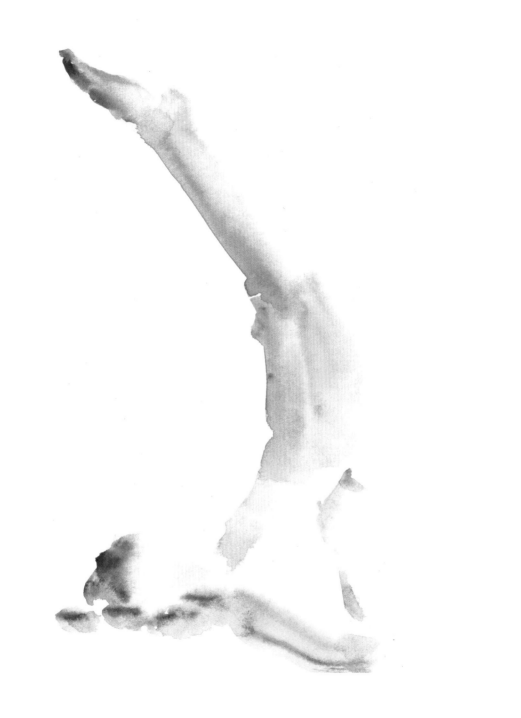

Throat proposals

A1 | Standing with feet parallel.

Let your arms hang down your front with one hand on top of the other.

Look down at your hands, letting them rise above your head as you inhale.

Follow the movement with your eyes.

Exhale, bringing your arms down again.

Follow the movement of your hands with your eyes.

Repeat these movements, listening attentively to the sound of your breath inside your throat.

A2 | Lying on your back.

Bend your knees up, keeping your feet parallel.

Place your arms and hands crossed behind your head on the floor.

Let your head rest on your arms like a pillow.

Listen to your breath as it moves down your throat towards your feet.

Rest and welcome the in-breath moving all the way into a very open throat.

After a few rounds of breath, release your arms and hands.

Re-cross them behind your head with the other hand on top and repeat the breaths.

A3   Lying on your back.

Bend your knees up, keeping your feet parallel on the ground.

Gradually shift the weight from your feet to your shoulders, lifting your back off the ground, while dropping and relaxing the back of the throat.

Exhale down to the soles of your feet for a few rounds.

Receive the inhalation into a very open throat.

A4 | Sitting in a comfortable position.

Touch the front of your throat with one hand and the back of your throat with the other.

Listen to the elasticity and flexibility of the throat as the air goes out and away from you … and as it comes back to you from a long distance.

After a few rounds of breath, release your legs and hands and change to the other side.

Then release your hands and stay listening to your breath inside your throat.

B1 | Standing with feet parallel.

Spread the soles of your feet on the ground.

Without resisting or imposing, follow the subtle shift of your body weight backwards and forwards.

Slow down your breath until it sounds even and smooth.

B2 | On all fours.

Root your hands and knees to the ground.

Encourage the exhalation to slide from the back of your throat to your tail.

Relax your ankles and feet.

Rest and let the inhalation move up the front from the tip of your tail to your throat.

B3   Lying on your back.

Bend your knees up, keeping your feet parallel on the ground.

Relax your arms and hands by the side of your body.

Visualise your exhalation sliding down the back of your throat, the back of your heart, the back of your navel.

Rest.

Visualise your inhalation climbing up and touching the front of your navel, the front of your heart and the front of your throat.

Stay with this circle until it becomes clear and smooth.

Throat proposals in daily life

While standing:
Keeping your feet parallel, spread the soles of your feet on the ground.

Follow, without resisting, the subtle shift of your body weight, backwards and forwards.

Slow down your breath so it sounds even and smooth in the passage of the throat.

While sitting:
Exhale and let your chin drop down slowly.

Pause.

As you inhale, gradually lift your head up.

While lying on your back:
Bend your knees up, keeping your feet parallel on the ground.

Relax your arms and hands by the side of your body.

Listen to your breath.

Be aware of the resemblance of your breath to the sound of waves breaking and receding on the shore.

The eyebrow centre
as captivating as a smile

The natural inclination of the whole body for harmony takes you by the hand and fulfils this inner wish by uncovering forgotten corners and hidden places.

As the whole organism is gradually placed back into its fruitful co-habitation with earth and space, the special areas of the body become aware of and exposed to the two elements. They are awakened and reborn.

From the feet, through the root, and via the tail, the back of the navel softens, the heart brightens, the throat rests and then these awakenings drift up to the centre of the eyebrows.

The undulation the body provides while searching for a harmonious alignment opens an inner path. The ripples will move towards the space between the eyes and will reverberate in the back of the skull.

The integration of neck and head into this wave that pervades the whole being requires time, as resistance in this part of the body is usually stronger than in any other part.

The wish to control and direct the rest of the body from "up there" is deeply ingrained and overbearing. But the few seconds when the head and neck let go of their domineering attitude gives us a taste of incredible lightness and relief.

A smile is born and gently spreads out.

The aim of transforming the whole being into a hollow green bamboo cane feels closer and more tangible.

Eyebrow centre proposals

A1 | Lying on your back.

Bend your knees up, keeping your feet parallel on the ground.

Bring your hands to your eyebrow centre, massaging and releasing.

Use your fingertips to smooth over the wrinkles on your forehead.

Massage your temples with circular movements, clockwise and anti-clockwise.

Gently touch the front and the back of your ears.

Slowly move down to massage your chin.

Rest your arms and hands by the side of your body and shift your attention to the air moving in and out of your nostrils.

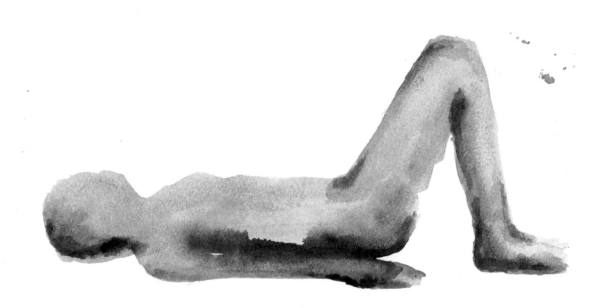

A2 | Lying on your front.

With your forehead on the ground, place your arms above your head.

Bring your attention to the whole length of your spine.

Follow your exhalation as it rolls down and touches each and every vertebra.

Observe the weight of your body moving down towards your pelvis and legs.

Rest and welcome the inhalation in.

As you exhale, the upper part of your spine becomes weightless, ready to elongate and float up.

Bring your elbows towards your chest and rest on the lower part of the arms – from the elbows to the fingertips.

Dropping your elbows into the ground, stay in this position for a few rounds of breath.

Exhaling, follow the breath going down from the back of your skull all the way to your feet, encouraging your forehead and eyes to smile.

After a few rounds of breath, gently move back onto your knees and heels.

Rest your forehead on your two fists which are placed one above the other on the floor.

Let your pelvis drop down towards your heels.

Rest for a few rounds of breath.

A3 | Standing with your back one metre away from a wall.

With feet parallel, let your arms hang down your front with one hand on top of the other.

Look at your hands and slowly bring them up while inhaling and down while exhaling.

Keep watching your hands until the movement is smooth with no interruptions.

Slowly, slowly, as you elongate your spine, your fingertips will touch the wall behind.

After a few rounds of breath, rest in a forward bend, releasing your arms, hands and head.

A4 | Sitting on your heels.

Look down to the ground, close your eyes and rest your gaze for a few minutes.

As you inhale, slowly open your eyes, move your head upwards and bring your gaze as high as is comfortable.

As you exhale, slowly lower your gaze and move your head down again until your eyes are closed.

Feel the movement getting easier and more harmonious.

A5 | Sitting on your heels.

Exhale towards your sitting bones and drop them.

Rest and welcome the inhalation in.

With an exhalation, cross your arms at the elbows with your hands in front of your eyebrow centre.

Extend your hands and cross them as well, the fingers of the lower hand are touching the palm of the upper one.

Breathe for a few rounds of breath.

Release your hands and arms, rest and play with crossing your elbows and hands the other way around.

B1 | Standing with feet parallel.

Shift your attention to the right foot.

Balance on it, lifting the left foot off the ground.

Extend your right arm above your head and oscillate gently to improve your equilibrium.

Listen to your breath and adjust and follow the pull that comes from gravity.

Become increasingly aware of the weight and rooting of the lower part of the body, while from the waist up, the body is light and extended.

Place both feet back on the ground, and then play with balancing on the other foot.

B2   Standing with your back one metre away from a wall.

With your feet parallel and both arms up, breathe down to the soles of your feet.

Feel your heels dropping, tail swinging, back of the navel wide and open.

Feel your heart softening, your throat relaxing and your head adjusting as it follows the movement.

Keep playing with this undulation as you exhale and inhale.

Improve your balance by looking far into the distance.

Without introducing any effort, keep growing and maybe touch the wall behind with your fingertips.

After a few rounds of breath, rest your upper back and arms by bending forwards.

B3 | Sitting on your heels.

Bring both your hands to the eyebrow centre, massaging and opening it.

Go down your nose to open your nostrils and cheekbones too.

Release your hands and bring your left hand into the right armpit.

Rest your right hand and wrist on your right thigh.

Exhale and feel the pull around your pelvis and legs.

Give in to it and rest at the end of the exhalation.

As you inhale, experience the lightness and elongation of your spine.

Stay with this breathing for a few rounds, becoming increasingly aware of your nostrils dilating as the air goes out and comes in.

After a few rounds, rest your arms and hands.

Change to the other side with your right hand in the left armpit, observing the breath as you breathe out and in through open nostrils.

Finish with your two arms crossed over your chest and your hands inside the opposite armpits, and stay like this for a few minutes.

Eyebrow centre proposals in daily life

While standing or while sitting:
Bring your hands to the eyebrow centre and massage this area,
trying to flatten out your wrinkles.

Draw your eyebrows apart lengthening them toward the temples
a few times.

While sitting on your heels:
Exhale from the nostrils and watch your exhalation moving in
spirals as far as the horizon. Relax your ankles and soften your
eyes to receive the in-breath coming from the horizon and into
your nostrils in spirals.

The crown of the head

breath after breath after breath

The rooting of the feet into the earth is the first conscious recognition of an outside friend.

It is a declaration of belonging that simultaneously awakens the natural urge to evolve upwards.

In this unfolding of depth and width, our body is taken along a cleverly laid-out map.

What we call discoveries are, in fact, the uncovering of forgotten and dusty places that become vivid and bright again.

So it is with the crown of the head.

The inner space at the top of the skull will widen and open only when the whole connection from the ground links upwards: the root, tail, navel, heart, throat and eyebrow centre.

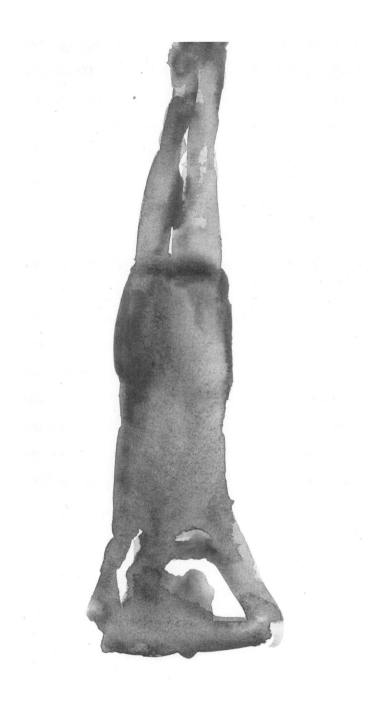

Crown proposals

The crown of the head is now open to a free dialogue with the vast and infinite space above.

To be welcomed by the space above is like meeting a friend who lives just around the corner. There is amazement and joy, but also regret for having been so out of touch.

The unfolding and exposure of the crown of the head permeates the whole standing posture with a sense of bliss.

Like a spring of boundless freedom that can, unexpectedly, express itself fully.

A1 | Lying on your back.

Bend your knees up, keeping your feet parallel on the ground.

Bring both your hands to the eyebrow centre.

Slowly move them up along the central line of the forehead and up and over your skull until you reach the top of your spine at the back of your neck.

Repeat this movement a few times.

Then place your two hands on the top of your skull with fingertips touching.

Slowly let your hands slide down the sides of your head to encourage more space between the two halves of the skull.

Let your arms and hands rest.

Exhale and let one leg rest on the floor.

With another exhalation, let the other leg rest as well.

Exhale backwards from the eyebrow centre, to the crown of the head and to the tip of the spine.

Rest.

Inhale from the tip of your spine to the crown of the head and forward to the eyebrow centre.

Repeat for a few rounds of breath and rest.

A2 | Lying on your back.

Bend your knees up, keeping your feet parallel on the ground.

One by one, bring your arms above your head and let them rest on the floor.

With an exhalation, extend your legs, one by one, on the ground.

Become aware of how the ground is touching your back, awakening each and every part of your body, and supporting it.

Exhale from the tips of your fingers, through the crown of your head, down the whole length of your body towards your heels.

Rest and welcome the inhalation coming in from your feet and heels, up the back of your body, through the crown of your head, to your fingertips.

Stay listening to the awakening of your back – its length and width – for a few rounds of breath.

A3 | Standing with your back one metre away from a wall.

With feet parallel, bring one arm to the back of your waist and raise the other one above your head.

Exhale down the back of your body as far as the heels, which roll on the floor, bringing an undulation to the whole body.

Pause and breathe in all the way up to your fingertips.

Keep elongating with the help of the breath until there is an opening on the crown of the head and the tips of your fingers gently touch the wall behind you without leaning on it.

After a few rounds of breath, exhale the upper part of your body into a forward bend.

Release your arms and feel the crown of the head opening.

Slowly roll back up to standing.

After a few rounds of attentive breath, release your arms and do the same on the other side.

A4 | Sitting on your heels.

Exhale from the crown of the head down the back of your spine.

Relax your sitting bones, knees, ankles and feet.

Be open to receiving the in-breath all the way up to the crown of your head.

Stay with this breath for a few rounds.

A5 | Sitting on your heels.

Exhale from the crown of the head, through your inner space to your two sitting bones.

Let them drop at the very end of the exhalation.

The inhalation comes in as a spring of water, enters your body and surges up to the top of your head like a fountain.

Play with this image for a few rounds of attentive breath.

End the practice with an easy, round, natural breathing.

B1 | Standing with your back one metre away from a wall.

With feet parallel, bring both arms above your head, and with the help of the right hand, open the left hand, wrist, elbow and armpit.

Let this ripple open as far as the hip, knee, ankle and centre of your foot at the left side.

Visualise the exhalation moving from the palm of your left hand as it streams down towards the centre of the left foot.

Let your body adjust and drop your heels.

Open your left side to receive the inhalation all the way from the left foot to the tips of the fingers on your left hand – which elongate.

Stay with this opening and releasing of the left side, inviting it to open more and elongate further for a few rounds of breath.

Rest your arms and legs and go through the same rhythm on the right side of your body.

Then bring both arms above your head.

Exhale from the palms of both hands to the soles of your feet.

Drop your heels and let your body fluctuate between the earth and space, freely back and forth, elongating without haste.

Maybe, after a few rounds of breath, your hands will touch the back wall and slide a bit further down without leaning on it.

B2 | Standing with feet parallel.

Elongate your body upwards, unfolding from the palms of your hands to the soles of your feet.

Feel the full length of your body, looking for more freedom and expansion.

Exhale, bending your upper back forwards.

Walk your hands, one hand at a time, forward on the floor, extending the spine as you do so.

Your head is relaxed and the crown of the head opens.

Walk your hands away from your feet and back again a few times.

Walk your hands back to your feet, exhaling as you roll your back up to standing again.

Stay standing for a few quiet breaths feeling long, open and extended.

B3 | Sitting cross-legged.

Be aware of the space between your two sitting bones.

When you exhale from the crown of the head, let your breath touch the tip of your spine, the back of your throat, the back of your heart, the back of your navel, tail and the root of your being.

Pause there and rest.

Enjoy the natural pause and witness the journey of the in-breath as it rises up from the root of your being to the front of your tail, the front of your navel, your heart, your throat and your eyebrow centre to the top of your head.

Pause and rest, letting the crown of the head clear, blossom and unfold.

Exhale again, down through the back of your body.

Rest and inhale up the front again, the breath touching each and every place along the way.

Stay and witness the journey of your breath for a few rounds.

Complete the practice with an exhalation through the root of your being.

Crown proposals in daily life

While standing:
Open your feet and spread the soles into the earth.

Simultaneously unfold and expose the crown of the head to the space above.

While sitting:
Be aware of your two sitting bones dropping at the end of your exhalation. Inhaling, let the breath move towards the crown of your head, from within.

While lying on your back:
Exhale to the soles of your feet. Drop the weight of your whole body into the ground.

Inhale very slowly through the whole length of your body to the crown of the head.

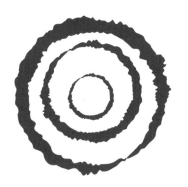

chapter four

Tangible benefits

Tangible benefits

To nurture and revitalise the special areas we have uncovered and awakened, here are some further explorations which can be practised daily.

Two practices that carry a deep invitation to approach the body as a whole.

They should be practised separately and repeated until the organism feels their benefits in a tangible way.

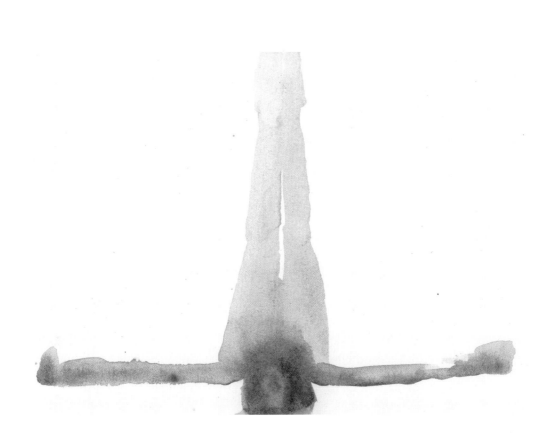

Weeding the path

Standing with feet parallel.

Find the central spot in between your two feet and feel the connection between the root of your being and this spot on the ground.

Breathe along this imaginary thread for a few breaths.

Place one hand on your tail and the other above your pubic bone. Feel the space cluttered with sodden earth, and the breath bringing back light and clarity as it moves in and out.
Exhale and inhale along this passage for a few breaths.

Move your hands and place one on your navel area and the other at the back of your waist. Feel the space in between your two hands and breathe. Feel the resistance of the weeds to be uprooted and the constant gentle breeze that will remove them. Exhale and inhale for a few breaths.

Place one hand on your heart area and the other in between your shoulder blades. Feel the passage as an overgrown path and the breath sweeping away the weeds.

Exhale and inhale for a few breaths.

Move your hands to the front and back of your throat. Feel the connection between these two points and let your breath sweep. Feel the breath as a breeze that removes withered flowers and clears the passage.

Exhale and inhale for a few breaths.

Move your hands to the eyebrow centre and the tip of the spine at the back of the skull. Feel the distance between your two hands and let yourself feel the breath reopening the path as it lifts and blows away the leaves fallen on it.

Exhale and inhale for a few breaths.

Bring your attention to the crown of your head, softening and exposing it to the space above. Connect with the space above and breathe up and down an invisible thread.

Exhale and inhale for a few breaths.

Gently and slowly move down from the crown of your head to the root of your being and the ground below, breathing for a few breaths in each and every place.

Finish the practice with a few natural and easy breaths.

At home

Lying on your back.

Let your body rest on the ground with the arms alongside your body and the legs wide apart.

Be open enough to receive the pull of gravity and let your exhalation roll down the full length of your body towards your feet like unravelling a thread.

Rest and welcome the in-breath.

Guide the next exhalation towards the centre of your pelvic floor and let it elongate as far as possible, away from your body. Inhale back along the same path.

Breathe along this imaginary coil for a few breaths.

Move your attention to the pubic bone and your tail. Discover the passage that connects these two places.

Let your breath clean and dust the passage, with the help of spiralling breath.

Shift your attention to the navel area and the back of the waist.

Polish this passage with spinning breath, allowing these circular air movements to clear and remove sediment along this path.

Move your attention to the heart area and the area in between your shoulder blades.

Let your breath be like a vortex that cleans and dusts this passage.

Shift your attention to the front and back of your throat. Feel the connection between these two places and let your breath, moving in spirals, sweep it and air it.

Move your attention to the eyebrow centre and the tip of your spine at the back of the skull.

Feel the passage that unites these two places and let the whirlpool of your breath purify it.

Bring your attention to the crown of the head, unfolding it and connecting it with the space around you. Breathe out and in, with spiralling motions clearing this opening.

Gently and slowly move down, with your attention and spiralling breath, from the crown of the head to the root of your being, pausing for a few breaths in each and every place.

Finish the practice with a few rounds of natural and quiet breath.

At the end

The students are lying on their backs.

Their spines are resting.

In a few moments, they will roll onto one side and sit up.

A different kind of silence enters the room and we smile at one another.

Palms of the hands are put together in gratitude.

There is a sense of bliss – we have been riding through waves that have brought us all to a peaceful shore.

There is a unique togetherness that comes from having been immersed in a timeless space and place.

We have been exploring the possibility of rooting and expanding at the same time. And our capacity to mould and change shape when connected to earth and sky.

The journey has been gradual.

We have taken it step by step with infinite time.

There is a sense of fulfilment as a primal need has been answered, a vital necessity has been met.

The room is vibrant.

About the authors

Sandra Sabatini started to study yoga in Florence with Dona Holleman. Some years later she met Vanda Scaravelli and began a journey under her guidance which has not ended.

In 1986 Sandra was invited to London by Mary Stewart to show her many pupils the approach Vanda had developed in teaching yoga. 'No ambition and infinite time', she often repeated, to keep the practice utterly simple. Later, in retreats offered by Thich Nhat Hanh, Sandra discovered the walking meditation again which Vanda had practised all along the road to Fiesole, and brought this into her practice.

For more than forty years Sandra has been teaching in Germany, the UK, Finland, Israel and most recently in India. She is the author of *Breath, Like a Flower* and co-author of *Autumn Winter Spring Summer*.

She lives in Campiglia in Tuscany where she holds residential courses. www.sandrasabatini.info

Michal Havkin was born in Jerusalem and lives in Tel-Aviv, Israel. She discovered yoga after more than 30 years of dancing professionally and teaching Modern Dance in Israel and abroad.

Her yoga practice consists of slow, gentle movements, connected to the breath and the space around us, and integrated with her extensive study of Buddhism and Feldenkrias technique. Michal has been studying and co-teaching with Sandra Sabatini for more than 18 years.

"My yoga practice," says Michal, "is about undoing, letting go, releasing, opening and softening with the wish to be quiet, to listen."

About the artist

Orly Maiberg is a graduate of the New York School of Visual Arts and lives and works in Tel Aviv. Her works were featured in numerous solo and group exhibitions in Israel, Europe and the USA.

She is represented by Noga Gallery. www.orlymaiberg.com

Notes

Also from YogaWords

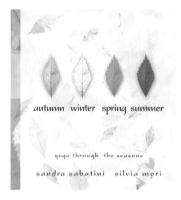

Awakening the Spine
Vanda Scaravelli

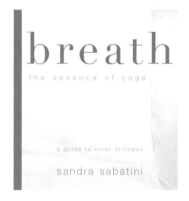

Autumn Winter Spring Summer
Sandra Sabatini & Silvia Mori

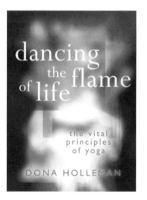

Breath
Sandra Sabatini

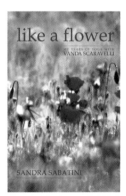

Like a Flower
Sandra Sabatini

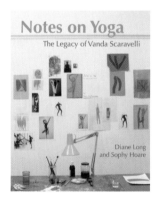

Notes on Yoga
Diane Long & Sophy Hoare

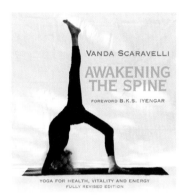

Dancing the Flame of Life
Dona Holleman

pinterandmartin.com/yogawords

YOGAWORDS